Cannabis Cookbook

GW01072047

DELICIOUS ASSORTMENT OF RECIPES FOR CANNABIS INFUSED FOOD, DESSERT, AND EXTRACTS!

TABLE OF CONTENTS

The Basics

(Recipes to bring your weed into a useable, cookable form)

Infused Olive Oil

Ingredients:

16oz Extra virgin olive oil

16g marijuana, decarbed and ground fine

Directions:

-Heat olive oil in a Crock Pot or in covered stove pot on medium/low heat. Avoid high temperatures.

-Add marijuana, let it simmer.

-Let oil cool for 1-3 hours, depending on the temperature. The oil should turn a darker brown color indicating is has absorbed the cannabis.

-Let cool

INFUSED COCONUT OIL

Serves: 16

Time: 120 Minutes

Ingredients:

8 oz coconut oil

8 g kief (or 16g shake)

Directions:

-Use a Crock Pot or use a stove top with a covered pot.

-Put all ingredients in pot and cook on medium heat for 1 hour up to 3 hours, never to exceed 260 degrees.

-Strain. Chill oil solution in your fridge overnight and allow to separate.

Cannabis Honey

Serves: 80 to 100

Time: 6 to 24 hours

Ingredients:

1 ounce cannabis

5 lbs (10 cups) honey

cheesecloth

string

Directions:

-Wrap cannabis in cheese cloth. Secure bundle with string.

-Place bundle in crock pot. Pour honey to cover.

-Cover and cook on low for 4 to 5 hours, stirring a few times per hour.

-Turn crock pot off and let honey sit to cool for up to 24 hours.

-Remove bundle from the honey, squeezing as much honey from the cheesecloth as possible.

-Ladle honey into jars to store.

Cannabis Butter

Ingredients:

1/4 ounce cannabis flowers, dried and finely ground

1/2 cup (one stick) unsalted butter

4 cups of water

Directions:

-Bring water to a boil in pan.

-Once boiled, melt butter in water

-Once the butter has melted, add the dried cannabis, while stirring to avoid clumping. Once weed is added into the saucepan, reduce heat to a very low simmer.

-Continue to simmer for about 2 1/2 to 3 hours or until the top of the water becomes much darker and thickens.

-Once the cannabis butter mixture has finished simmering, secure several layers of cheesecloth around the opening of your storage container with a rubber band, leaving a bit of slack in the middle of the container.

-Slowly pour the cannabis butter mixture through a strainer

-Once all of the cannabis butter has been poured into the container, carefully remove the cheesecloth. Wrap the strained weed into a ball inside the cheesecloth, then use your spoon to squeeze out any remaining liquid.

-Let the cannabis butter mixture cool for 30 minutes to an hour

-Place mixture in your refrigerator for 6 to 8 hours, or until solid

CANNABIS MAYO

Serves: 16

Time: 10 Minutes

Ingredients:

2 cups Infused Olive Oil

4 egg yolks

1 Tbsp Dijon

1 tsp vinegar

1 Tbsp hot water

Directions:

-The easiest way to complete this task is with a blender or food processor

-Mix all ingredients together in a blender and blend until desired consistency

Optional: If you don't have a blender, a bowl and a whisk can be used as plan B

TINCTURE

Ingredients:

45 g marijuana

750 ml Everclear or glycerin

Directions:

-Decarb cannabis and grind into a powder.

-Use a funnel to transfer ground cannabis into a clear 1.75 ml bottle and pour 750ml of Everclear over cannabis.

-Screw on the top and shake vigorously 3 times a day for 30 days.

Breakfast

MUFFINS

Serves: 4

Time: 20 minutes

Ingredients:

½ cup 100 percent vegetable oil

6 grams ground cannabis or three grams full melt hash (no straining necessary)

½ a cup water

Blueberries

Cake Flour

Directions:

-In a mixing bowl, add cake mix and slowly pour Cannabis oil into it. Add three eggs. Pour the mixture into a mixer and blend well. Run the mixer at a low speed to avoid the formation of air pockets. Add the blueberries and fold them in such a way that they don't break. Continue adding blue berries till the colour of the mix changes slightly

-Once the blueberries are folded in well, scrape the bowl down and add the mixture to muffin cups. Using two spoons, transfer the mix to the cups, ensuring that they are only ¾ full. Keep the cups on a tray and transfer the tray to a pre-heated oven. Bake the muffins at 350 degrees for about 20 minutes. Halfway through the baking process, spin the tray through 180 degree so that all the muffins are warmed to the same temperature.

-At the end of 20 minutes, take the tray out, cool the muffins and have a nice time eating them. Check out the video below for a step by step visual walkthrough of the previous steps.

Yogurt Parfait

Serves: 4

Prep: 8 Minutes

Ingredients

2 cups Yogurt

1 cup berries, fresh

1 cup Marmalade, Blueberry and Raspberry are favorites

1/2 cup Weed Honey

1 cup Granola (optional)

Directions:

-Grab a glass and layer the berries, marmalade, honey, yogurt, and granola.

As a tip: use a to-go cup. The transportability of this parfait nice and it is a great way to balance your metabolism for a great day outside.

COFFEE

Ingredients:

1 liberal pinch of pounded hash

4 tsp of finely pulverised Arabian mocha

2 pinches crushed nutmeg

2 pinches crushed cinnamon

1 full pot of freshly made coffee

Sugar

Milk or Creamer

Directions:

-First of all brew your coffee just the way you would do usually in your coffee pot.

-Put in all the ingredients on the recipe into the coffee- you may add more or less hash as you prefer. Add the mixture into a coffee pot.

-Then, place the pot on a low flame allowing it to come to a boil.

-When the mixture starts to boil, remove the pot from the flame. Add some cream, sugar and enjoy a beautiful morning

FLAX SEED OMELETTE

Ingredients:

3 eggs

1 tsp Cannabis Butter

1 tsp Infused Coconut Oil

4 oz mixed veggies

2 oz mushrooms

1 oz pepitas

1 tsp flax seed

Directions:

-In an 8 inch non stick frying plan add the fat and heat to Medium-High.

-Whip eggs and season with salt and pepper.

-Pour in eggs and start forming the base with a rubber spatula, add remaining ingredients.

BISCUITS

Ingredients:

3/4 cup of mashed sweet potato (1 large sweet potato)

1/2 or 1/3 cup milk

1 and 1/2 cup all-purpose flour

2 Tbsp sugar

1 Tbsp baking powder

1 tsp salt

6 Tbsp of cold unsalted cannabis butter

Directions:

-The first step is to heat your oven to 425 degrees Fahrenheit and greasing a biscuit sheet or tray. Then peel and chop the sweet potato to boil it. Once it has cooked through mash it up and let cool for some time. Once the sweet potato mash has cooled down add 1/3 cup of milk to it and whisk it together.

-Next mix the dry ingredients namely flour, sugar, baking powder and salt in a bowl and keep it aside. Cut 6 tablespoons of the cannabis butter into smaller pieces and add it to the dry ingredients mixture. Using knife, fork or biscuit cutter cut the cannabis butter into the mixture until you get a crumbly mealy mixture.

-After this add the sweet potato mash and milk mixture to the cannabis butter and flour mixture and fold it in gently. If you feel that mix is too dry you can add some more milk to get a better consistency for the mix.

-Now that the dough is ready it can be rolled out. Sprinkle some dry flour on to a clean work surface and put the dough on it. Then roll out the dough using a rolling pin to your desired thickness. Now that the dough is rolled out use a biscuit cutter or glass or bottle lid to cut out the biscuits into simple discs. Keep repeating this process till the entire dough is used up.

-Next place the biscuit discs on the biscuit tray or sheet and put them in the preheated oven to cook for about 12 to 15 minutes till they rise to look golden brown and are firm to the touch. That's how easy it is to make yummy crunchy sweet potato marijuana biscuits at home. You may add a touch of honey cannabis butter on top of the biscuits to make them extra tasty and gooey.

GREEK OMELETTE

Serves: 1

Time: 10 Minutes

Ingredients:

3 eggs

1 tsp Cannabis Butter

1 tsp Infused Olive Oil

3 oz grilled chicken, shredded

1 oz feta

1 oz grape tomatoes

1 Tbsp chopped olives

1 tsp fresh oregano

1 oz green onion

2 oz sour cream

Directions:

-First, create a mix of chicken and veggies in one bowl and a mix of seasoned whipped eggs in a separate bowl.

-Heat a saute pan on medium high heat and pour in your seasoned eggs.

-Stir your eggs for about 30 seconds and smooth out.

-Place chicken and filling inside your omelet and fold in half.

-Cook for a minute or so on each side.

WAFFLES

Serves: 4

Time: 15 minutes

Ingredients:

1/2 gram BHO Shatter

2 Tbsp coconut oil

1/2 lb of bacon

2 eggs

1/2 cup grated cheese

One cup pancake waffle mix of your choice

3/4 cup milk

Directions:

-Place the double boiler on the heat with water below and coconut oil on top. Melt coconut oil in a double boiler till it melts completely. Now add BHO concentrate till it is completely incorporated into the oil. This will ensure that the marijuana is bycarboxylated to make it effective. Remove from the heat and place in a mixing bowl till cool.

-Fry the bacon till it is nice and crispy. Cool and chop into bits. Keep aside. Mix two eggs into the mixing bowl that has the coconut oil and BHO. Whisk lightly, pour in the milk and whisk again till all the ingredients are incorporated. Add the one cup of pancake and waffle mix and whisk thoroughly. Once mixed well add cheese and the bacon bits and again mix till fully incorporated.

-Heat the waffle iron to medium high heat. Measure out half a cup of the mix and place in the heated waffle iron. Smoothen quickly and close the cover. Remove when browned. You will know it's done once the steam comes out the sides and the cheese begins to trickle out. Make sure you remove it only when it is browned to ensure the marijuana is decarboxylated so you get the kick. This mixture will make four waffles if you use half a cup at a time

FRENCH TOAST

Serves: 4

Time: 30 Minutes

Ingredients:

1 French baguette

1 and ½ Tbsp butter

3 Tbsp canna butter

4 eggs

1 cup milk

¼ cup sugar

3 Tbsp maple syrup

1 tsp vanilla extract

½ tsp salt

powdered sugar

Directions:

-Lightly butter the baking dish. Cut the baguette crosswise at an angle to make 8 pieces. Each slice should be at least ¾ inches thick. Keep aside. In a small bowl cream the two kinds of butters till they are thoroughly combined. Now spread this butter on one side of each of the 8 slices. Now arrange these 8 slices, butter side up, into the greased baking dish.

-In a separate mixing bowl add the eggs, milk, maple syrup, sugar, vanilla and salt. Whisk the ingredients till they blend. Pour this mixture over the bread and allow the slices to soak it up by pressing it down on it with a spoon. Cover the dish and refrigerate for 8 hours.

-When you wish to have your Baked Marijuana French Toast, preheat the oven to 350°F. Once heated uncover the dish and place the baking tray in the oven and bake for 45 minutes or until the tops turn golden brown. Dust them with powdered sugar and enjoy the power

Snacks

PEANUT BUTTER

Ingredients:

A small bowl or ramekin

A measuring spoon

A regular spoon

Directions:

-In this recipe we are making cannabis peanut butter for a single serving. For the first step, measure out one and a half teaspoons of cannabis oil and pour it into the ramekin. The quantity of cannabis oil can vary up to 2 teaspoons depending on how much peanut butter you put it in later. Make sure you use non- GMO oil as it is much healthier. You can leave the cannabis buds in the oil if you don't mind the taste and texture of it.

-Next, measure 2 tablespoons of peanut butter and put it in with the cannabis oil in the ramekin. You should preferably use high fructose corn syrup free peanut butter. You can use chunky or creamy peanut butter according to your taste. Mix the peanut butter and cannabis oil together well using a spoon. Once you get a smooth and creamy consistency your cannabis peanut butter is done. It won't be too sticky or slimy. Spread it on a slice of bread and you are good to go! You will get a nice hit from the cannabis in the peanut butter.

-If you want this cannabis peanut butter to be thicker, just put it in the fridge for half an hour and it will be the perfect consistency. The peanut butter masks the flavour of the cannabis and makes a great start for the day with breakfast.

CRAB CAKES

Serves: 4

Time: 25 minutes

Ingredients:

1 cup celery or sweet corn

1/2 cup roasted bells, chives, parsley

1/2 - 1 cup Cannabis Mayo

1/4 Cup Dijon

2 Tbsp Siracha

2 Tbsp Tarragon

2 lb shelled cooked crab

1 lb panko

Directions:

-Mix all ingredients except the crab and panko.

-Once combined, fold in the crab to the mix and 1 cup of panko.

-Season with salt, pepper and celery seed if you fancy.

-Refrigerate for 2 hours.

BRUSCHETTA

Ingredients:

3/4 cup Cannabis Oil

Pot Pesto

One loaf ciabatta

8 tomatoes

3 Tbsp brown sugar

1 clove garlic minced

Balsamic vinegar

1 teaspoon Dijon mustard

Salt

Pepper

Onion powder

Directions:

-Slice the ciabatta and arrange the sliced ciabatta on a baking sheet on a tray. Now brush each slice with THC oil. Put the oiled ciabatta slices into the oven for 3 minutes at 350°F. Baking adds an extra zing to the flavor so don't forget this important step. After three minutes remove from the oven and place sliced tomato pieces on top of the ciabatta. Three tomato pieces a slice is ideal. Add more if you like tomatoes. Bake again for another 5 minutes at 350°F.

-While the ciabatta and the tomatoes are in the oven take a mixing bowl. Add brown sugar minced garlic, Dijon mustard, onion powder, salt and pepper to taste to the mixing bowl. Whisk the ingredients till smooth. Once smooth add the balsamic vinegar and the THC oil to the mixture and whisk again till all the ingredients combine together. Your balsamic vinaigrette is now ready. Take out the tomatoes from the oven after 5 minutes are up. Now drizzle some balsamic vinaigrette on top of the tomatoes and then add a tablespoon of pot pesto right on top. Your Kind Bud Bruschetta is ready to eat. Serve warm

Twice Baked Potato

Ingredients:

4 large potatoes

1 Tbsp light brown sugar

1/4 cup sour cream

1/4 cup Cannabis Butter

salt and pepper to taste

bacon bits (optional)

scallions (optional)

cheese (optional)

Directions:

-Preheat oven to 375 degrees.

-Place potatoes on a baking sheet and bake until tender (about an hour.

-Remove from oven and allow the potatoes to cool.

-Cut off the top of each potato, lengthwise.

-Scoop out the insides while making sure the skin still holds its shape.

-Mix the scooped potato bits, sour cream, Cannabis Butter, salt and pepper together in a medium mixing bowl. Mix until very smooth.

-Scoop the potato mixture back into the potato skins.

-Bake in oven for 10 minutes or until tops begin to brown.

-Add toppings as desired.

Beef Jerky

Ingredients:

3 lbs of cheap steak.

2 Tbsp Black pepper

1/8 of weed (broken up)

Salt to taste

Directions:

-Shred the steak with the hand and remove all the bones. Place the weed, steak, pepper and salt inside the bag and shake it up thoroughly so that the beef is well coated.

-Place the bag inside the dehydrator for 3 to 36 hours depending on how soft or tough you like the jerky to be.

-Remove and eat strips of the jerky to get your full enjoyment. The jerky will last a week. This jerky is also being commercially made as a snack because it is so delicious

.

DILL PICKLE DIP

Ingredients:

1 cup Cannabis Mayo

2 egg whites, chopped

1/4 cup capers rinsed, minced

1/4 cup cornichons, chopped

3 shallots, chopped

3 cloves roasted garlic, chopped

½ bunch tarragon, chopped

1 Tbsp red wine vinegar

1 lemon, zest, juice

Directions:

-In a large mixing bowl mix everything together and season with salt and pepper

GUACAMOLE

Serves: 10

Time: 1 hour

Ingredients:

4 ripe avocados, peeled

1 cucumber, peeled and chopped

½ cup green onions, chopped

2 cloves of garlic, minced

1 jalapeno pepper

½ cup Cannabis oil

Juice of 2 limes

1 tsp salt

Directions:

-Get your food processer ready to operate.

-Put the peeled and sliced avocados into your blender.

-Follow it up by adding the chopped cucumber and then the jalapeno pepper. Then put in the chopped green onions.

-Next, add the lime juice and ½ a cup of THC oil and top it all with a bit of salt.

-Blend to desired consistency

-Pour out the mixture into the glass bowl

-Serve

Dinner

Burgers

Serves: 6

Time: 30 minutes

Ingredients:

2/3 to one pound of ground beef or turkey

Approximately .7 to 1 gram of weed, cleaned and ground into a powder (if it is good and dry it is much easier)

Salt & Pepper (or any preferred seasonings to add flavor)

Directions:

-Since making a hamburger is a pretty basic task you really don't have to deviate much from the traditional methods of making one. Making sure you get your weed evenly dispersed throughout the meat is the most important part, and after much trial and error an effective method has been achieved.

-First, take your meat and flatten it into a large circle on a clean counter-top or cutting surface. Flatten it out evenly making sure the thickness of the meat is fairly consistent.

-Now take your powdered pot and sprinkle it over the surface of the meat; you want the weed to cover the top of the meat entirely.

-Now fold the meat over, completely enclosing the pot inside. At this point you will begin to need and work the meat to make sure the weed is evenly distributed throughout.

-Next you want to make your patty or patties. Shape and form them into just what you want size and shape wise or just make one great big one to satisfy that monstrous appetite.

-Season the patty or patties using salt, pepper, garlic (fresh or powdered), and any others you like. Feel free to experiment, and keep in mind that the weed will add seasoning as well.

-Grill or fry for 5 or 6 minutes per side (or to preferred temperature)

-Eat it on a bun or bun-free with your favorite garnishments

CHILI

Serves: 14

Time: 120 Minutes

Ingredients:

1 red, yellow, white onion, small dice

2 red, yellow, green bell peppers, small dice

6 garlic cloves, minced

6 Tbsp Infused Olive Oil

1 lb ground meat of your choice

2 cups cooked kidney beans, drained

2 cups cooked pinto beans, drained

2 cups crushed fire roasted tomatoes

6 oz tomato paste

2 tsp paprika, chili powder

1 tsp cayenne pepper

Directions:

-To start, simply add non medicated olive oil to stock pot and brown meat of your choice,

-Once browned, drain in a colander

-Add medicated oil to stock pot and add veggies and season with salt and pepper.

-Add tomato paste and cook for 5-8 minutes.

-Add remaining ingredients and let simmer until it tastes just right.

Pizza

Serves: 1

Time: 20 minutes

Ingredients:

1/4 tsp weed

1 slice of cooked pizza

Directions:

-Simply reheat already-cooked pizza in the microwave and you will be able to mix the weed with the cheese fat and for a sufficiently short duration to avoid vaporizing more cannabinoids.

-Take the pizza slice and sprinkle the weed on it as though you were sprinkling oregano. Make sure that you take off the toppings temporarily so that the weed is directly on top of the cheese. Heat the slice of pizza in the microwave for around 20 to 30 seconds depending on the thickness of the crust or till the cheese just about melts. Enjoy!

STRIP STEAK

Ingredients:

4 Prime Strips

1 Cup Cannabis Butter or Olive Oil

Directions:

-Season the steaks with medicated Olive Oil or Cannabis Butter and some salt and pepper.

-Leave them out at room temperature for 30 minutes prior to cooking.

-Heat your grill to high for 15 minutes before grilling.

-Grill steaks until desired doneness, flipping the steaks every 2 minutes.

-Allow meat to rest for 6 minutes after cooking.

Optional: Spoonful of Cannabis Butter can be melted on top of the Steak for an extra high and great taste

Mac n Cheese

Ingredients:

1/2 cup of unsalted butter

1/2 cup of cannabis butter

2 tsp of salt

1 tsp of black pepper

1/2 a tsp of cayenne pepper

1 cup of grated cheddar cheese

1 cup of grated Mozzarella cheese

1 cup of grated Swiss cheese

3/4 cup of grated Parmesan cheese

1 cup of flour

3/4 cup of bread crumbs

4 cups of milk

1 pound of cooked macaroni pasta

Directions:

-Heat the unsalted regular butter and the cannabis butter in a deep pan and let them melt well for 3 to 5 minutes. Once they have melted, add the flour in little by little, whisking it in with the butter properly.

-Next, add the milk in small batches just like the flour and whisk it in as well to form a smooth mixture. If you add the milk all together at once the mixture will become lumpy. Once you are done mixing in the milk, add the different seasonings namely, salt, black pepper and cayenne pepper.

-After seasoning take the pan off the heat to add the various cheeses namely, cheddar cheese, Swiss cheese, Mozzarella cheese and Parmesan. Start by adding the cheddar a little bit at a time and mix it in nicely. Continue the same process with the other three cheeses in the order of Swiss, Mozzarella and Parmesan. Don't add all of the Parmesan, leave some aside.

-Now that you've got your cheese sauce to the right creamy consistency, you can add the cooked pasta to the sauce and mix it in well with a spatula. Shift this mac and cheese mixture into a greased oven baking dish. Mix the Parmesan cheese that you left aside with some cannabis butter and bread crumbs and sprinkle it on top of the mac and cheese mixture.

-Next, put the baking dish in the oven at 350 degrees Fahrenheit for 30 to 40 minutes to cook. Once the crust of the mac and cheese has turned golden brown you can take it out of the oven and voila!

WATERMELON SALAD

Ingredients:

1 watermelon

4 oz feta, crumbled

1 oz fresh mint, chopped

1 tsp cayenne

1 tsp smoked salt

1 oz Infused Olive Oil

1 ea grapefruit, juiced

Directions:

-In a small mixing bowl whisk together medicated olive oil and citrus juice.

-Next add the salt and cayenne pepper.

-Toss in your watermelon and mint and put it on a plate.

-Garnish with the crumbled Feta.

CHICKEN ALFREDO

Serves: 4

Time: 55 Minutes

Ingredients:

1 lb fresh Potsta, cooked

1 lb grilled chicken, bite size

1/2 lb Brocolli Florettes, cooked

1/4 Cup all-purpose flour

1 small onion, minced

4 garlic cloves, minced

2 Tbsp Infused Olive Oil

1 cup Cannabis Cream

1 cup Parmesan cheese

1 cup favorite other cheese

2 cups Chicken Stock

2 Tbsp Cannabis Butter

Directions:

-In a medium sauce pot heat Infused Olive Oil and cook down onions until they are translucent.

-Once you can almost see through them, add the garlic cook for 2 minutes.

-Toss the flour into the pot and stir with a wooden spoon for 2-3 minutes.

-Slowly add the Cannabis Cream and stock alternatively to form a nicely thickened emulsified sauce.

-Start to add the grated cheeses and finish with tablespoon or two of Cannabis Butter.

-Combine remaining ingredients and enjoy!

Drinks

MARGARITAS

Ingredients:

Four fresh limes

Jar of honey

Several cups of ice cubes

Infused medicated tequila

Margarita glasses

High-powered blender

Grater

Salt, preferably sea salt (optional)

Directions:

-Place 1-2 cups of ice cubes in blender.

-Scrape 4-8 tablespoons of honey (warming the honey slightly in the microwave can make it easier to pour and distribute) into the blender along with the ice.

-Squeeze 2-3 large limes for their juice, and add the resulting juice to the mixture in the blender. Free-pour in the alcohol to reach the level of strength you desire in your margarita. Blend sufficiently until smooth.

-Chill margarita glasses while mixing. Once they are chilled, remove from refrigerator and begin to garnish.

-Dampen and dip the rims in salt if a salted rim is desired. Slice the fourth lime into thin half-slices, and put a small notch in the flesh of each slice so that it can be easily slipped over the rim of the glass.

-Distribute margarita mixture into glasses and grate a small amount of lime zest over the top of each portion. Enjoy while they are still frosty!

SOUR DIESEL

Ingredients:

2 oz Pisco

1 oz fresh lime juice

1 oz glycerin Tincture

1 egg white

1 dash Amargo bitters

Directions:

-Add the Pisco, lime, Tincture and egg white to a shaker with NO ice.

-Shake 10 to 12 seconds.

-Add ice and shake 30 seconds

-Pour and strain into an old fashioned cocktail glass.

-Add dash of bitters to garnish.

Marijuana Milkshake

Ingredients:

1 part of Crème de cacao

2 parts of Midori which is a Japanese melon liqueur

1 part of Half and half cream

Ice cubes

Directions:

-Put some ice cubes into the drinks shaker and add the crème de cacao, Midori and half and half cream in the proportions mentioned under ingredients.

-Shake the drinks shaker well and pour the milkshake into a regular glass or a shot glass and your marijuana milkshake is ready to be enjoyed!

Tequila Sunrise

Serves: 1

Ingredients:

1 1/2 oz Infused tequila

3/4 Cup Orange Juice

A few ice cubes

1 Tbsp grenadine syrup

1 slice orange, for garnish

1 maraschino cherry for garnish

Directions:

-Shake Tequila and OJ.

-Pour over ice.

-Float the Grenadine.

-Garnish

MARIJUANA MOJITOS

Ingredients:

2 ounces of marijuana rum

Fresh mint leaves

2 tsp of white sugar

Two fresh limes

A dash of bitters

Ice cubes

A bottle of club soda

Directions:

-First, add a teaspoon of sugar to each of the glasses. Then cut the lime in half and using the squeezer squeeze the lime juice of half a lime into each of the glasses. You can use the juice of half a lime to a full lime depending on the size of the glass you are using. For this recipe we are using medium sized glasses.

-Next, add a dash of the bitters to each of the glasses. After this add a few (3 to 4) fresh mint leaves to the mixture in the glasses and using the wooden pestle carefully muddle or crush the mint leaves with the mixture of sugar, lime juice and bitters in each of the glasses.

-Now, add a few (2 to 3) ice cubes to each glass and pour an ounce of marijuana rum each into the two glasses. Top off the mojito cocktail mixture in the glasses with club soda to the brim, add a cool straw to each glass and your home made marijuana mojitos are ready to be enjoyed!

Dessert

CARAMEL

Ingredients:

1 cup cannabis butter

2 1/4 cup brown sugar

dash of salt

1 cup light corn syrup

1 (14 oz.) can sweetened condensed milk

1 tsp. vanilla

Directions:

-Melt butter; add brown sugar and salt.

-Stir until combined.

-Stir in light corn syrup.

-Gradually add milk; stir constantly.

-Cook and stir over med heat, until candy reaches firm ball stage (245F), about 12 to 15 min.

-Remove from heat; stir in vanilla, pour into 9″ by 13″ pan.

-Cool, cut and wrap.

Chocolate Chip Cookies

Ingredients:

1 1/3 cup of flour

1/3 cup of sugar

2/3 cup of brown sugar

1/2 cup of cannabutter

1 1/3 cup of chocolate chips

1/4 tsp of baking soda

1/4 tps of salt

2 tsp of vanilla extract

1 egg

Directions:

-The first step is to pre-heat your oven to 325 degrees and grease the baking sheet that you will be using. Grab a medium sized bowl and combine the 1 1/3 cups of all purpose natural flour, 1/4 tablespoon of baking soda and 1/4 tablespoon of salt. Whisk this mixture until everything is combined and the set it aside for the time being. Grab another medium sized bowl and mix the 1/2 cup of cannabis butter, 1/3 cup of granulated sugar and 2/3 cups of packed brown sugar. For the best results, use a mixer. Continue mixing until the contents in this bowl are creamy.

-Once the mixture is all set, add in the 2 teaspoons of vanilla extract and egg. Continue mixing with your hand mixture until the butter/sugar/brown sugar combination has a light consistency, and then add in the chocolate chips. Once the chocolate chips are added, gently stir in the flower mixture from the first bowl into the second. It may take awhile, but continue mixing until you have decent looking and firm cookie dough.

-Once the dough is ready, you will then spoon the mixture out into 1/4 cup cookies on a sheet and spread them out accordingly. Place them into the preheated oven at 325 degrees and let the cookies bake for 18-25 minutes. Remove the sheet from the oven when the cookies are a crisp golden brown and let them cool for approximately 10-15 minutes before removing from the sheet. Once the cookies have cook, sit down and enjoy your hard work!

Classic Brownies

Serves: 12

Time: 70 Minutes

Ingredients:

1 2/3 cups granulated sugar

3/4 cup baking cocoa

1 1/3 cups all-purpose flour

1/2 tsp baking powder

1/4 tsp salt

2 large eggs

2 Tbsp water

3/4 cup Cannabis Butter, melted

2 tsp vanilla extract

Directions;

-Preheat your oven to 350°F

-Grease your baking pan with the non-stick spray

-Mix the cannabis butter, sugar, cocoa, flour, baking powder, and salt in your mixing bowl

-Next, add the water. You'll want to be pouring slowly and whisking quickly to remove any lumps.

-Once all of the water is added to the mixture, add the eggs and finally the vanilla extract.

-When your batter is well-mixed, pour it evenly into your baking pan and pop it in the oven.

-Bake for somewhere between 18 to 25 minutes. It can vary on a lot of things, but the toothpick test is the best way to tell if it's done.

-Let cool and enjoy

POPSICLES

Serves: 5

Time: 1 Hour

Ingredients:

2 mangos, you will want these to be peeled, and you will want to flesh to be chopped into chunks

2 cups of your favorite vanilla yogurt

4 Tbsp of cream of coconut

2-3 Tbsp of Infused Coconut Oil

3 Tbsp coconut sugar

2 tsp coconut extract

If you do not like the taste of coconut, then you are more than welcome to use any substitute.

Directions:

-There are actually only four easy steps you need to follow to get yourself on your way to enjoying your popsicles, and those are as follows

-Place all of your ingredients into your blender

-To puree them until they are smooth.

-Pour them into Popsicle molds and then

-Freeze them.

Cinnamon Chocolate Bark

Servings: 15

Time: 10 Minutes

Ingredients:

1 lb chocolate

1 tsp cinnamon

1 tsp sea salt

1 range, zest

2 broken candy canes

Directions:

-Line a sheet pan with a Silpat and heat some water for a double boiler.

-Melt the chocolate in a bowl over boiling water and stir in cinnamon.

-Spread Mexican Chocolate mixture over Silpat and grate orange over top

APPLE PIE BARS

Servings: 12

Time: 40 Minutes

Ingredient:

1/2 Cup Cannabis Butter at room temperature

3/4 Cup sugar

2 eggs

1 tsp vanilla

1 1/2 Cup flour

3/4 tsp baking powder

1 tsp apple pie spice

2 Cup apple pie filling

Directions:

-Cream butter; add sugar and beat well. Beat in eggs one at a time. Add vanilla.

-Gradually stir in sifted dry ingredients.

-Spread ¾ of dough in a lightly grease 8x11 inch baking pan.

-Spread apple pie filling over dough.

-Spoon remaining dough over pie filling, spreading lightly. (Not all pie filling will be covered.)

-Bake at 375 degrees for 35-40 minutes.

BUTTER CAKE

Ingredients:

1 cup Cannabis butter, room temp

1 1/2 cup sugar

3 large eggs

3 egg yolks

2 Tbsp vanilla

3 1/2 cups cake flour

1 Tbsp baking powder

1/2 tsp salt

1 ea lemon, zest and juice

10 fl.oz milk room temp

Directions:

-In a fresh bowl, with a mixer on medium-high speed (use the paddle attachment if using a standing mixer), beat butter and sugar until fluffy and pale yellow, 4 to 5 minutes. Add eggs, then yolks, one at a time, beating well after each addition and scraping down sides of bowl as necessary. Beat in vanilla, lemon zest and juice.

-In another bowl, mix flour, baking powder, and salt. Stir (or beat at low speed) about a third of the flour mixture into butter mixture. Stir in half the milk just until blended. Stir in another third of the flour mixture, then remaining milk, followed by remaining flour. Scrape batter equally into two buttered and floured 9-inch round cake pans and spread level, or one 9 x 13 pan, buttered and floured.

-Bake in a 350° regular or convection oven until a wooden skewer inserted in the center comes out clean, 25 to 30 minutes. Cool on racks in pans for 10 minutes, then invert cakes onto racks and remove pans. Cool completely before frosting.

Printed in Poland
by Amazon Fulfillment
Poland Sp. z o.o., Wrocław